GW00361532

This Keto Diet Journal

Belongs To:

_____

Yearly Keto Day Tracker

	JAN	FEB	MAR	APR	MAY	JUN	JUL	AUG	SEP	OCT	NOV	DEC
1												
2												
3												
4												
5												
6												
7												
8												
9												
10												
11												
12												
13												
14												
15												
16												
17												
18												
19												
20												
21												
22												
23												
24												
25												
26												
27												
28												
29												
30												
31												

COLOR IN THE DAYS THAT YOU WERE IN KETOSIS TO KEEP TRACK OF YOUR WEIGHT LOSS PROGRESS!

NOTES & REFLECTIONS:

TOTAL DAYS IN KETOSIS:

30 Day Keto Challenge

WHY THIS GOAL MEANS SO MUCH

MY PLAN OF ACTION

- [ ]
- [ ]
- [ ]
- [ ]
- [ ]
- [ ]
- [ ]
- [ ]
- [ ]
- [ ]
- [ ]
- [ ]
- [ ]
- [ ]
- [ ]
- [ ]
- [ ]

INSPIRATIONAL REMINDERS

STARTED >

FINISHED >

1	2	3	4	5	6	7	8	9	10
11	12	13	14	15	16	17	18	19	20
21	22	23	24	25	26	27	28	29	30

30-DAY KETO RESULTS

PERSONAL ACCOMPLISHMENTS

Keto Before & After

WEIGHT	WEIGHT
BMI	BMI
BODY FAT	BODY FAT
MUSCLE	MUSCLE
CHEST	CHEST
WAIST	WAIST
HIPS	HIPS
THIGHS	THIGHS
CALF	CALF
BICEP	BICEP
OTHER :	OTHER :
OTHER :	OTHER :

Weight Loss *Tracker*

MONTHLY GOAL

DATE:

BUST				
WAIST				
HIPS				
BICEP				
THIGH				
CALF				
WEIGHT				
TOTAL WEIGHT LOSS >>				

Macro Quick Reference

MACRO TRACKER

QTY	TYPE	PROTEIN	FAT	CARBS	CALS	NOTES

Weight Loss *Start Date*

Outline your most important fitness goals

Describe how you see yourself in six months

DATE	KETO WEIGHT LOSS ACTION PLAN	PERSONAL MILESTONES

Ketogenic Foods

MEATS	VEGGIES	VEGGIES	FRUITS
Beef	Avocado	Cucumber	Blackberries
Sausage	Asparagus	Chards	Cranberries
Bacon	Argula	Bell Peppers	Blueberries
Lamb	Broccoli	Green Beans	Lemon
Pork	Cauliflower	Collards	Lime
Veal	Brussel Sprouts	Mushrooms	Raspberries
Chicken/Turkey	Cabbage	Spinach	Strawberries
Eggs	Celery	Olives	Plantains (paleo)

DAIRY	CONDIMENTS	OILS & FATS	HERBS & SPICES
Cheese (all kinds)	Balsamic Vinegar	Avocado Oil	Garlic
Sour Cream	Beef/Chicken Broth	Butter	Salt & Pepper
Cream Cheese	Bonito Flakes	Coconut Butter	Oregano
Heavy Cream	Tartar Sauce (keto)	Duck Fat	Paprika
Greek Yogurt	Dijon Mustard	Lard/Ghee	Cumin
Almond Milk	Mayo	Nut Oils	Chili Pepper
Cashew Milk	Low Sugar Ketchup	Olive Oil	Basil
Coconut Cream	Pickles	Pork Rinds	Ginger

BAKING	FISH/SEAFOOD	DRINKS	MISC.
Almond Flour	Anchovy	Diet Soda (moderation)	Canned Tuna
Almond Meal	Haddock / Cod	Coffee	Pesto
Cashew Flour	Halibut	Tea	Soy Sauce
Oat Fiber	Crab/Lobster	Gatorade Zero	Aioli
Psyllium Husk	Mackerel	Protein Shake	Béarnaise
Whey Protein	Salmon	Club Soda	Vinaigrette
Flax meal	Tuna	Broth	Hot Sauce
Hazelnut Flour	Red Snapper	Coconut Water	Guacamole

NOTES:

Keto Friendly Foods

KETO FRIENDLY FOODS	NET CARBS	PROTEINS	FAT

FOODS TO EAT IN MODERATION	NET CARBS	PROTEINS	FAT

Low Carb Grocery Ideas

FRESH PRODUCE

☐	Asparagus	☐	Cauliflower	☐	Onions
☐	Avocado	☐	Celery	☐	Radishes
☐	Bell Peppers	☐	Cucumber	☐	Salad Mix
☐	Berries	☐	Eggplant	☐	Squash
☐	Broccoli	☐	Fennel	☐	Tomatoes
☐	Brussel Sprouts	☐	Garlic	☐	Bok Choi
☐	Cabbage	☐	Green Beans	☐	Chives
☐	Carrots	☐	Mushrooms	☐	Spinach

MEAT AND SEAFOOD

☐	Bacon	☐	Lamb	☐	Fish
☐	Beef	☐	Pork	☐	Crab
☐	Bison	☐	Rotisserie Chicken	☐	Lobster
☐	Chicken	☐	Sausage	☐	Scallops
☐	Deli meat	☐	Turkey	☐	Shrimp
☐	Ground Beef / Ground Turkey	☐	Oyster	☐	Mussels

DAIRY PRODUCTS

☐	Butter	☐	Eggs	☐	Sour Cream
☐	Cheese	☐	Greek Yogurt, full fat	☐	Ghee
☐	Cream Cheese	☐	Heavy Whipping Cream	☐	Mayo

PANTRY ITEMS

☐	Avocado oil	☐	Tea/Coffee	☐	Moon Cheese
☐	Beef Jerky	☐	Pork Rinds	☐	Low Carb Protein Bars
☐	Bone Broth	☐	Mayonnaise	☐	All Natural Peanut Butter
☐	Tuna, Salmon (canned)	☐	Low Carb Salad Dressing	☐	Stevia
☐	Coconut Butter	☐	Olive oil, extra virgin	☐	Almonds
☐	Coconut Oil	☐	Olives	☐	Spices
☐	Almond Milk	☐	Sweeteners	☐	Almond Flour

FROZEN / OTHER

☐		☐		☐	
☐		☐		☐	
☐		☐		☐	
☐		☐		☐	

Low Carb Shopping List

FRESH PRODUCE

MEAT AND SEAFOOD

DAIRY PRODUCTS

PANTRY ITEMS

FROZEN / OTHER

Meal Planner

WEEK OF

GROCERY LIST

- ☐
- ☐
- ☐
- ☐
- ☐
- ☐
- ☐
- ☐
- ☐
- ☐
- ☐
- ☐
- ☐
- ☐
- ☐
- ☐
- ☐

MON

TUES

WED

THUR

FRI

SAT

SUN

Weight Loss *Journal*

MONDAY

TUESDAY

WEDNESDAY

THURSDAY

FRIDAY

SATURDAY

SUNDAY

WEEK OF:

DATE	WEIGHT LOSS ACTION PLAN

NOTES

My Weight Loss Routine

CREATING A ROUTINE FOR SUCCESS

WEIGHT LOSS SUCCESS: HABIT & ROUTINE TRACKER

DRINK LOTS OF WATER TODAY	TRACK TOTAL CARB INTAKE

COMPLETE TOP 3 GOALS OF THE DAY

1

2

3

PLAN MY MEALS FOR THE DAY:

BREAKFAST	LUNCH	DINNER

DAILY TRACKER & TO DO LIST	ACCOMPLISHMENTS

NOTES

Daily Tracker

SLEEP TRACKER:

DATE _____

☼ RISE: _____   🌙 zᶻz BEDTIME: _____   💭 SLEEP (HRS): _____

NOTES FOR THE DAY

_____

_____

_____

EXERCISE / WORKOUT ROUTINE

TOP 6 PRIORITIES OF THE DAY

○ _____   ○ _____

○ _____   ○ _____

○ _____   ○ _____

IN A STATE OF KETOSIS?

YES   NO   UNSURE

WATER INTAKE TRACKER

DAILY ENERGY LEVEL

HIGH	**MEDIUM**	**LOW**

BREAKFAST

FAT: CARBS: PROTEIN: CALORIES:

LUNCH

FAT: CARBS: PROTEIN: CALORIES:

DINNER

FAT: CARBS: PROTEIN: CALORIES:

SNACKS

FAT: CARBS: PROTEIN: CALORIES:

END OF THE DAY TOTAL OVERVIEW

CARBS   FAT   PROTEIN
CALORIES

Staying On Track

MY WEIGHT LOSS DIARY:

_____

_____

_____

_____

WATER TRACKER

〇 〇 〇 〇 〇 〇 〇 〇

LOW CARB SNACKS

NOTES & REMINDERS

_____

_____

_____

_____

_____

_____

_____

_____

_____

DOODLE MY MOOD

BREAKFAST IDEAS

LUNCH IDEAS

DINNER IDEAS

Daily Tracker

SLEEP TRACKER:

DATE _____

RISE: _____   BEDTIME: _____   SLEEP (HRS): _____

NOTES FOR THE DAY

_____

_____

_____

EXERCISE / WORKOUT ROUTINE

TOP 6 PRIORITIES OF THE DAY

- ⚪ _____   ⚪ _____
- ⚪ _____   ⚪ _____
- ⚪ _____   ⚪ _____

IN A STATE OF KETOSIS?

YES   NO   UNSURE

WATER INTAKE TRACKER

DAILY ENERGY LEVEL		
HIGH	**MEDIUM**	**LOW**

BREAKFAST

FAT: CARBS: PROTEIN: CALORIES:

LUNCH

FAT: CARBS: PROTEIN: CALORIES:

DINNER

FAT: CARBS: PROTEIN: CALORIES:

SNACKS

FAT: CARBS: PROTEIN: CALORIES:

END OF THE DAY TOTAL OVERVIEW

CARBS   FAT   PROTEIN
CALORIES

Staying On Track

MY WEIGHT LOSS DIARY:

WATER TRACKER

LOW CARB SNACKS

NOTES & REMINDERS

DOODLE MY MOOD

BREAKFAST IDEAS

LUNCH IDEAS

DINNER IDEAS

Daily Tracker

SLEEP TRACKER:

DATE _____

☀ RISE: [   ]   🌙 BEDTIME: [   ]   ☁ SLEEP (HRS): [   ]

NOTES FOR THE DAY

....

....

....

EXERCISE / WORKOUT ROUTINE

TOP 6 PRIORITIES OF THE DAY

- ● .... ● ....
- ● .... ● ....
- ● .... ● ....

IN A STATE OF KETOSIS?

YES   NO   UNSURE

WATER INTAKE TRACKER

DAILY ENERGY LEVEL

HIGH	MEDIUM	LOW

BREAKFAST

FAT: CARBS: PROTEIN: CALORIES:

LUNCH

FAT: CARBS: PROTEIN: CALORIES:

DINNER

FAT: CARBS: PROTEIN: CALORIES:

SNACKS

FAT: CARBS: PROTEIN: CALORIES:

END OF THE DAY TOTAL OVERVIEW

CARBS   FAT   PROTEIN
CALORIES

Staying On Track

MY WEIGHT LOSS DIARY:

_____

_____

_____

_____

WATER TRACKER

LOW CARB SNACKS

NOTES & REMINDERS

DOODLE MY MOOD

BREAKFAST IDEAS

LUNCH IDEAS

DINNER IDEAS

Daily Tracker

SLEEP TRACKER:

DATE _____

☼ | RISE: | 🌙 zᶻᶻ | BEDTIME: | ☁️zᶻᶻ | SLEEP (HRS):

NOTES FOR THE DAY

_____

_____

_____

EXERCISE / WORKOUT ROUTINE

TOP 6 PRIORITIES OF THE DAY

○ _____ ○ _____

○ _____ ○ _____

○ _____ ○ _____

IN A STATE OF KETOSIS?

YES   NO   UNSURE

WATER INTAKE TRACKER

DAILY ENERGY LEVEL		
HIGH	**MEDIUM**	**LOW**

BREAKFAST

FAT: CARBS: PROTEIN: CALORIES:

LUNCH

FAT: CARBS: PROTEIN: CALORIES:

DINNER

FAT: CARBS: PROTEIN: CALORIES:

SNACKS

FAT: CARBS: PROTEIN: CALORIES:

END OF THE DAY TOTAL OVERVIEW

CARBS   FAT   PROTEIN
CALORIES

Staying On Track

MY WEIGHT LOSS DIARY:

WATER TRACKER

LOW CARB SNACKS

NOTES & REMINDERS

DOODLE MY MOOD

BREAKFAST IDEAS

LUNCH IDEAS

DINNER IDEAS

Daily Tracker

SLEEP TRACKER:

DATE _____

☀ | RISE: | 🌙 zzz | BEDTIME: | 💤 zZZ | SLEEP (HRS):

NOTES FOR THE DAY

_____

_____

_____

IN A STATE OF KETOSIS?

YES   NO   UNSURE

WATER INTAKE TRACKER

EXERCISE / WORKOUT ROUTINE

DAILY ENERGY LEVEL

HIGH	**MEDIUM**	**LOW**

BREAKFAST

FAT: CARBS: PROTEIN: CALORIES:

LUNCH

FAT: CARBS: PROTEIN: CALORIES:

DINNER

FAT: CARBS: PROTEIN: CALORIES:

SNACKS

FAT: CARBS: PROTEIN: CALORIES:

TOP 6 PRIORITIES OF THE DAY

- ● _____ ● _____
- ● _____ ● _____
- ● _____ ● _____

END OF THE DAY TOTAL OVERVIEW

CARBS CALORIES	FAT	PROTEIN

Staying On Track

MY WEIGHT LOSS DIARY:

_____

_____

_____

_____

WATER TRACKER

◊ ◊ ◊ ◊ ◊ ◊ ◊ ◊

LOW CARB SNACKS

NOTES & REMINDERS

_____

_____

_____

_____

_____

_____

_____

_____

_____

DOODLE MY MOOD

BREAKFAST IDEAS

LUNCH IDEAS

DINNER IDEAS

Daily Tracker

SLEEP TRACKER:

DATE _____

 RISE: BEDTIME: 🌙 SLEEP (HRS):

NOTES FOR THE DAY

_____

_____

_____

EXERCISE / WORKOUT ROUTINE

TOP 6 PRIORITIES OF THE DAY

- ⦾ _____
- ⦾ _____
- ⦾ _____

IN A STATE OF KETOSIS?

YES   NO   UNSURE

WATER INTAKE TRACKER

DAILY ENERGY LEVEL

HIGH	MEDIUM	LOW

BREAKFAST

FAT: CARBS: PROTEIN: CALORIES:

LUNCH

FAT: CARBS: PROTEIN: CALORIES:

DINNER

FAT: CARBS: PROTEIN: CALORIES:

SNACKS

FAT: CARBS: PROTEIN: CALORIES:

END OF THE DAY TOTAL OVERVIEW

CARBS   FAT   PROTEIN
CALORIES

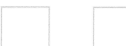

Staying On Track

MY WEIGHT LOSS DIARY:

_____

_____

_____

_____

WATER TRACKER

NOTES & REMINDERS

DOODLE MY MOOD

LOW CARB SNACKS

BREAKFAST IDEAS

LUNCH IDEAS

DINNER IDEAS

Daily Tracker

SLEEP TRACKER:

DATE _____

RISE: _____ ZzZ BEDTIME: _____ ZzZ SLEEP (HRS): _____

NOTES FOR THE DAY

_____

_____

_____

EXERCISE / WORKOUT ROUTINE

TOP 6 PRIORITIES OF THE DAY

- ⬤ _____   ⬤ _____
- ⬤ _____   ⬤ _____
- ⬤ _____   ⬤ _____

IN A STATE OF KETOSIS?

YES   NO   UNSURE

WATER INTAKE TRACKER

DAILY ENERGY LEVEL

HIGH   **MEDIUM**   **LOW**

BREAKFAST

FAT: CARBS: PROTEIN: CALORIES:

LUNCH

FAT: CARBS: PROTEIN: CALORIES:

DINNER

FAT: CARBS: PROTEIN: CALORIES:

SNACKS

FAT: CARBS: PROTEIN: CALORIES:

END OF THE DAY TOTAL OVERVIEW

CARBS   FAT   PROTEIN
CALORIES

Staying On Track

MY WEIGHT LOSS DIARY:

_____
_____
_____
_____

WATER TRACKER

◊ ◊ ◊ ◊ ◊ ◊ ◊ ◊

LOW CARB SNACKS

NOTES & REMINDERS

_____
_____
_____
_____
_____
_____
_____
_____
_____

DOODLE MY MOOD

BREAKFAST IDEAS

LUNCH IDEAS

DINNER IDEAS

Keto Go To Meals

BREAKFAST	LUNCH	DINNER	SNACKS
BREAKFAST	LUNCH	DINNER	SNACKS
BREAKFAST	LUNCH	DINNER	SNACKS
BREAKFAST	LUNCH	DINNER	SNACKS
BREAKFAST	LUNCH	DINNER	SNACKS
BREAKFAST	LUNCH	DINNER	SNACKS
BREAKFAST	LUNCH	DINNER	SNACKS

WEEK OF:

KETO *Meal* LOG BOOK

	BREAKFAST	LUNCH	DINNER	SNACKS
MONDAY				
TUESDAY				
WEDNESDAY				
THURSDAY				
FRIDAY				
SATURDAY				
SUNDAY				

Weekly Fasting *Tracker*

Week Of: _____

MONDAY

	12	1	2	3	4	5	6	7	8	9	10	11	12	1	2	3	4	5	6	7	8	9	10	11
Goal	12	1	2	3	4	5	6	7	8	9	10	11	12	1	2	3	4	5	6	7	8	9	10	11
Actual	12	1	2	3	4	5	6	7	8	9	10	11	12	1	2	3	4	5	6	7	8	9	10	11

TUESDAY

	12	1	2	3	4	5	6	7	8	9	10	11	12	1	2	3	4	5	6	7	8	9	10	11
Goal	12	1	2	3	4	5	6	7	8	9	10	11	12	1	2	3	4	5	6	7	8	9	10	11
Actual	12	1	2	3	4	5	6	7	8	9	10	11	12	1	2	3	4	5	6	7	8	9	10	11

WEDNESDAY

	12	1	2	3	4	5	6	7	8	9	10	11	12	1	2	3	4	5	6	7	8	9	10	11
Goal	12	1	2	3	4	5	6	7	8	9	10	11	12	1	2	3	4	5	6	7	8	9	10	11
Actual	12	1	2	3	4	5	6	7	8	9	10	11	12	1	2	3	4	5	6	7	8	9	10	11

THURSDAY

	12	1	2	3	4	5	6	7	8	9	10	11	12	1	2	3	4	5	6	7	8	9	10	11
Goal	12	1	2	3	4	5	6	7	8	9	10	11	12	1	2	3	4	5	6	7	8	9	10	11
Actual	12	1	2	3	4	5	6	7	8	9	10	11	12	1	2	3	4	5	6	7	8	9	10	11

FRIDAY

	12	1	2	3	4	5	6	7	8	9	10	11	12	1	2	3	4	5	6	7	8	9	10	11
Goal	12	1	2	3	4	5	6	7	8	9	10	11	12	1	2	3	4	5	6	7	8	9	10	11
Actual	12	1	2	3	4	5	6	7	8	9	10	11	12	1	2	3	4	5	6	7	8	9	10	11

SATURDAY

	12	1	2	3	4	5	6	7	8	9	10	11	12	1	2	3	4	5	6	7	8	9	10	11
Goal	12	1	2	3	4	5	6	7	8	9	10	11	12	1	2	3	4	5	6	7	8	9	10	11
Actual	12	1	2	3	4	5	6	7	8	9	10	11	12	1	2	3	4	5	6	7	8	9	10	11

SUNDAY

	12	1	2	3	4	5	6	7	8	9	10	11	12	1	2	3	4	5	6	7	8	9	10	11
Goal	12	1	2	3	4	5	6	7	8	9	10	11	12	1	2	3	4	5	6	7	8	9	10	11
Actual	12	1	2	3	4	5	6	7	8	9	10	11	12	1	2	3	4	5	6	7	8	9	10	11

Weekly Progress

Monday

Tuesday

Wednesday

Thursday

Friday

Saturday

Sunday

Notes

Low Carb Grocery Ideas

FRESH PRODUCE

☐ Asparagus	☐ Cauliflower	☐ Onions
☐ Avocado	☐ Celery	☐ Radishes
☐ Bell Peppers	☐ Cucumber	☐ Salad Mix
☐ Berries	☐ Eggplant	☐ Squash
☐ Broccoli	☐ Fennel	☐ Tomatoes
☐ Brussel Sprouts	☐ Garlic	☐ Bok Choi
☐ Cabbage	☐ Green Beans	☐ Chives
☐ Carrots	☐ Mushrooms	☐ Spinach

MEAT AND SEAFOOD

☐ Bacon	☐ Lamb	☐ Fish
☐ Beef	☐ Pork	☐ Crab
☐ Bison	☐ Rotisserie Chicken	☐ Lobster
☐ Chicken	☐ Sausage	☐ Scallops
☐ Deli meat	☐ Turkey	☐ Shrimp
☐ Ground Beef / Ground Turkey	☐ Oyster	☐ Mussels

DAIRY PRODUCTS

☐ Butter	☐ Eggs	☐ Sour Cream
☐ Cheese	☐ Greek Yogurt, full fat	☐ Ghee
☐ Cream Cheese	☐ Heavy Whipping Cream	☐ Mayo

PANTRY ITEMS

☐ Avocado oil	☐ Tea/Coffee	☐ Moon Cheese
☐ Beef Jerky	☐ Pork Rinds	☐ Low Carb Protein Bars
☐ Bone Broth	☐ Mayonnaise	☐ All Natural Peanut Butter
☐ Tuna, Salmon (canned)	☐ Low Carb Salad Dressing	☐ Stevia
☐ Coconut Butter	☐ Olive oil, extra virgin	☐ Almonds
☐ Coconut Oil	☐ Olives	☐ Spices
☐ Almond Milk	☐ Sweeteners	☐ Almond Flour

FROZEN / OTHER

☐	☐	☐
☐	☐	☐
☐	☐	☐
☐	☐	☐

Low Carb Shopping List

FRESH PRODUCE

MEAT AND SEAFOOD

DAIRY PRODUCTS

PANTRY ITEMS

FROZEN / OTHER

Meal Planner

WEEK OF

GROCERY LIST

- ☐
- ☐
- ☐
- ☐
- ☐
- ☐
- ☐
- ☐
- ☐
- ☐
- ☐
- ☐
- ☐
- ☐
- ☐
- ☐
- ☐

MON

TUES

WED

THUR

FRI

SAT

SUN

Weight Loss *Journal*

MONDAY

TUESDAY

WEDNESDAY

THURSDAY

FRIDAY

SATURDAY

SUNDAY

WEEK OF:

DATE	WEIGHT LOSS ACTION PLAN

NOTES

My Weight Loss Routine

WEIGHT LOSS SUCCESS: HABIT & ROUTINE TRACKER	
DRINK LOTS OF WATER TODAY	**TRACK TOTAL CARB INTAKE**

COMPLETE TOP 3 GOALS OF THE DAY

1
2
3

PLAN MY MEALS FOR THE DAY:

BREAKFAST	LUNCH	DINNER

DAILY TRACKER & TO DO LIST	ACCOMPLISHMENTS

NOTES

Daily Tracker

SLEEP TRACKER:

DATE _____

RISE: _____ | BEDTIME: _____ | SLEEP (HRS): _____

NOTES FOR THE DAY

_____

_____

_____

EXERCISE / WORKOUT ROUTINE

IN A STATE OF KETOSIS?

YES   NO   UNSURE

WATER INTAKE TRACKER

DAILY ENERGY LEVEL

HIGH	MEDIUM	LOW

BREAKFAST

FAT: CARBS: PROTEIN: CALORIES:

LUNCH

FAT: CARBS: PROTEIN: CALORIES:

DINNER

FAT: CARBS: PROTEIN: CALORIES:

SNACKS

FAT: CARBS: PROTEIN: CALORIES:

TOP 6 PRIORITIES OF THE DAY

END OF THE DAY TOTAL OVERVIEW

CARBS   FAT   PROTEIN
CALORIES

Staying On Track

MY WEIGHT LOSS DIARY:

_____
_____
_____
_____

WATER TRACKER

NOTES & REMINDERS

_____
_____
_____
_____
_____
_____
_____
_____
_____
_____
_____
_____

DOODLE MY MOOD

LOW CARB SNACKS

BREAKFAST IDEAS

LUNCH IDEAS

DINNER IDEAS

Daily Tracker

SLEEP TRACKER:

DATE _____

☀ RISE: [   ]   🌙 BEDTIME: [   ]   💭 SLEEP (HRS): [   ]

NOTES FOR THE DAY

_____
_____
_____

EXERCISE / WORKOUT ROUTINE

[   ]

TOP 6 PRIORITIES OF THE DAY

-
-
-
-
-
-

IN A STATE OF KETOSIS?

YES   NO   UNSURE

WATER INTAKE TRACKER

💧 💧 💧 💧 💧 💧 💧 💧

DAILY ENERGY LEVEL		
HIGH	**MEDIUM**	**LOW**

BREAKFAST

FAT: CARBS: PROTEIN: CALORIES:

LUNCH

FAT: CARBS: PROTEIN: CALORIES:

DINNER

FAT: CARBS: PROTEIN: CALORIES:

SNACKS

FAT: CARBS: PROTEIN: CALORIES:

END OF THE DAY TOTAL OVERVIEW

CARBS   FAT   PROTEIN
CALORIES

[   ]   [   ]   [   ]   [   ]

Staying On Track

MY WEIGHT LOSS DIARY:

_____

_____

_____

_____

WATER TRACKER

○ ○ ○ ○ ○ ○ ○ ○

LOW CARB SNACKS

NOTES & REMINDERS

_____

_____

_____

_____

_____

_____

_____

_____

_____

DOODLE MY MOOD

BREAKFAST IDEAS

LUNCH IDEAS

DINNER IDEAS

Daily Tracker

SLEEP TRACKER:

DATE _____

RISE: _____   BEDTIME: _____   SLEEP (HRS): _____

NOTES FOR THE DAY

_____
_____
_____

EXERCISE / WORKOUT ROUTINE

IN A STATE OF KETOSIS?

YES   NO   UNSURE

WATER INTAKE TRACKER

DAILY ENERGY LEVEL

HIGH	MEDIUM	LOW

BREAKFAST

FAT: CARBS: PROTEIN: CALORIES:

LUNCH

FAT: CARBS: PROTEIN: CALORIES:

DINNER

FAT: CARBS: PROTEIN: CALORIES:

SNACKS

FAT: CARBS: PROTEIN: CALORIES:

TOP 6 PRIORITIES OF THE DAY

END OF THE DAY TOTAL OVERVIEW

CARBS   FAT   PROTEIN
CALORIES

Staying On Track

MY WEIGHT LOSS DIARY:

_____

_____

_____

_____

WATER TRACKER

LOW CARB SNACKS

NOTES & REMINDERS

DOODLE MY MOOD

BREAKFAST IDEAS

LUNCH IDEAS

DINNER IDEAS

Daily Tracker

SLEEP TRACKER:

DATE _____

RISE: | BEDTIME: | SLEEP (HRS):

NOTES FOR THE DAY

_____

_____

_____

EXERCISE / WORKOUT ROUTINE

IN A STATE OF KETOSIS?

YES   NO   UNSURE

WATER INTAKE TRACKER

DAILY ENERGY LEVEL		
HIGH	**MEDIUM**	**LOW**

BREAKFAST

FAT: CARBS: PROTEIN: CALORIES:

LUNCH

FAT: CARBS: PROTEIN: CALORIES:

DINNER

FAT: CARBS: PROTEIN: CALORIES:

SNACKS

FAT: CARBS: PROTEIN: CALORIES:

TOP 6 PRIORITIES OF THE DAY

END OF THE DAY TOTAL OVERVIEW

CARBS   FAT   PROTEIN
CALORIES

Staying On Track

MY WEIGHT LOSS DIARY:

_____

_____

_____

_____

_____

WATER TRACKER

LOW CARB SNACKS

NOTES & REMINDERS

_____

_____

_____

_____

_____

_____

_____

_____

_____

_____

_____

DOODLE MY MOOD

BREAKFAST IDEAS

LUNCH IDEAS

DINNER IDEAS

Daily Tracker

SLEEP TRACKER:

DATE _____

RISE:	BEDTIME:	SLEEP (HRS):

NOTES FOR THE DAY

_____

_____

_____

EXERCISE / WORKOUT ROUTINE

IN A STATE OF KETOSIS?

YES   NO   UNSURE

WATER INTAKE TRACKER

DAILY ENERGY LEVEL

HIGH	**MEDIUM**	**LOW**

BREAKFAST

FAT: CARBS: PROTEIN: CALORIES:

LUNCH

FAT: CARBS: PROTEIN: CALORIES:

DINNER

FAT: CARBS: PROTEIN: CALORIES:

SNACKS

FAT: CARBS: PROTEIN: CALORIES:

TOP 6 PRIORITIES OF THE DAY

END OF THE DAY TOTAL OVERVIEW

CARBS CALORIES	FAT	PROTEIN

Staying On Track

MY WEIGHT LOSS DIARY:

_____

_____

_____

_____

WATER TRACKER

LOW CARB SNACKS

NOTES & REMINDERS

DOODLE MY MOOD

BREAKFAST IDEAS

LUNCH IDEAS

DINNER IDEAS

Daily Tracker

SLEEP TRACKER:

DATE _____

☀ | RISE: | | zᶻᶻ 🌙 | BEDTIME: | | zᶻᶻ ☁ | SLEEP (HRS): |

NOTES FOR THE DAY

_____

_____

_____

EXERCISE / WORKOUT ROUTINE

IN A STATE OF KETOSIS?

YES   NO   UNSURE

WATER INTAKE TRACKER

💧 💧 💧 💧 💧 💧 💧 💧

DAILY ENERGY LEVEL		
HIGH	**MEDIUM**	**LOW**

BREAKFAST

FAT: CARBS: PROTEIN: CALORIES:

LUNCH

FAT: CARBS: PROTEIN: CALORIES:

DINNER

FAT: CARBS: PROTEIN: CALORIES:

SNACKS

FAT: CARBS: PROTEIN: CALORIES:

TOP 6 PRIORITIES OF THE DAY

-
-
-

END OF THE DAY TOTAL OVERVIEW

| CARBS | FAT | PROTEIN |
CALORIES		

Staying On Track

MY WEIGHT LOSS DIARY:

_____

_____

_____

_____

WATER TRACKER

NOTES & REMINDERS

DOODLE MY MOOD

LOW CARB SNACKS

BREAKFAST IDEAS

LUNCH IDEAS

DINNER IDEAS

Daily Tracker

SLEEP TRACKER:

DATE _____

☼ RISE: _____   🌙 BEDTIME: _____   💤 SLEEP (HRS): _____

NOTES FOR THE DAY

IN A STATE OF KETOSIS?

YES   NO   UNSURE

WATER INTAKE TRACKER

💧 💧 💧 💧 💧 💧 💧 💧

EXERCISE / WORKOUT ROUTINE

DAILY ENERGY LEVEL		
HIGH	**MEDIUM**	**LOW**

BREAKFAST

FAT: CARBS: PROTEIN: CALORIES:

LUNCH

FAT: CARBS: PROTEIN: CALORIES:

DINNER

FAT: CARBS: PROTEIN: CALORIES:

SNACKS

FAT: CARBS: PROTEIN: CALORIES:

TOP 6 PRIORITIES OF THE DAY

END OF THE DAY TOTAL OVERVIEW

CARBS   FAT   PROTEIN
CALORIES

Staying On Track

MY WEIGHT LOSS DIARY:

_____

_____

_____

_____

WATER TRACKER

NOTES & REMINDERS

_____
_____
_____
_____
_____
_____
_____
_____
_____
_____
_____

DOODLE MY MOOD

LOW CARB SNACKS

BREAKFAST IDEAS

LUNCH IDEAS

DINNER IDEAS

Keto Go To Meals

FAVORITE KETO FRIENDLY MEALS

BREAKFAST	LUNCH	DINNER	SNACKS
BREAKFAST	LUNCH	DINNER	SNACKS
BREAKFAST	LUNCH	DINNER	SNACKS
BREAKFAST	LUNCH	DINNER	SNACKS
BREAKFAST	LUNCH	DINNER	SNACKS
BREAKFAST	LUNCH	DINNER	SNACKS
BREAKFAST	LUNCH	DINNER	SNACKS

KETO *Meal* LOG BOOK

	BREAKFAST	LUNCH	DINNER	SNACKS
MONDAY				
TUESDAY				
WEDNESDAY				
THURSDAY				
FRIDAY				
SATURDAY				
SUNDAY				

Weekly Fasting *Tracker*

Week Of: _____

MONDAY

Goal	12	1	2	3	4	5	6	7	8	9	10	11	12	1	2	3	4	5	6	7	8	9	10	11
Actual	12	1	2	3	4	5	6	7	8	9	10	11	12	1	2	3	4	5	6	7	8	9	10	11

TUESDAY

Goal	12	1	2	3	4	5	6	7	8	9	10	11	12	1	2	3	4	5	6	7	8	9	10	11
Actual	12	1	2	3	4	5	6	7	8	9	10	11	12	1	2	3	4	5	6	7	8	9	10	11

WEDNESDAY

Goal	12	1	2	3	4	5	6	7	8	9	10	11	12	1	2	3	4	5	6	7	8	9	10	11
Actual	12	1	2	3	4	5	6	7	8	9	10	11	12	1	2	3	4	5	6	7	8	9	10	11

THURSDAY

Goal	12	1	2	3	4	5	6	7	8	9	10	11	12	1	2	3	4	5	6	7	8	9	10	11
Actual	12	1	2	3	4	5	6	7	8	9	10	11	12	1	2	3	4	5	6	7	8	9	10	11

FRIDAY

Goal	12	1	2	3	4	5	6	7	8	9	10	11	12	1	2	3	4	5	6	7	8	9	10	11
Actual	12	1	2	3	4	5	6	7	8	9	10	11	12	1	2	3	4	5	6	7	8	9	10	11

SATURDAY

Goal	12	1	2	3	4	5	6	7	8	9	10	11	12	1	2	3	4	5	6	7	8	9	10	11
Actual	12	1	2	3	4	5	6	7	8	9	10	11	12	1	2	3	4	5	6	7	8	9	10	11

SUNDAY

Goal	12	1	2	3	4	5	6	7	8	9	10	11	12	1	2	3	4	5	6	7	8	9	10	11
Actual	12	1	2	3	4	5	6	7	8	9	10	11	12	1	2	3	4	5	6	7	8	9	10	11

Weekly Progress

Monday

Tuesday

Wednesday

Thursday

Friday

Saturday

Sunday

Notes

Keto 15 Task *Challenge*

1

CREATE A KETO
JOURNAL AND DOCUMENT
YOUR PROGRESS

COMPLETED ☐

2

CHOOSE 7 KETO FRIENDLY
RECIPES TO TRY

COMPLETED ☐

3

CREATE A WEEKLY
MEAL PLANNER

COMPLETED ☐

4

LOG EVERYTHING YOU EAT
IN A WEIGHT LOSS APP

COMPLETED ☐

5

PURCHASE A FOOD SCALE
AND SPIRALIZER

COMPLETED ☐

6

TRY BULLET PROOF
COFFEE

COMPLETED ☐

7

WEIGH YOURSELF
EVERY WEEK

COMPLETED ☐

8

GO ALCOHOL FREE FOR
ONE WEEK

COMPLETED ☐

9

TRY A 12-HOUR
INTERMITTENT FAST

COMPLETED ☐

10

CHECK AND LOG YOUR
BODY MEASUREMENTS

COMPLETED ☐

11

LIST ALL THE REASONS WHY
KETO WILL WORK FOR YOU

COMPLETED ☐

12

LEARN TO MAKE FAT BOMBS

COMPLETED ☐

13

MONITOR YOUR
WATER INTAKE

COMPLETED ☐

14

INCREASE YOUR HEALTHY
FAT INTAKE

COMPLETED ☐

15

TEST KETONE LEVELS
USING STRIPS

COMPLETED ☐

Low Carb Grocery Ideas

FRESH PRODUCE

☐	Asparagus	☐	Cauliflower	☐	Onions
☐	Avocado	☐	Celery	☐	Radishes
☐	Bell Peppers	☐	Cucumber	☐	Salad Mix
☐	Berries	☐	Eggplant	☐	Squash
☐	Broccoli	☐	Fennel	☐	Tomatoes
☐	Brussel Sprouts	☐	Garlic	☐	Bok Choi
☐	Cabbage	☐	Green Beans	☐	Chives
☐	Carrots	☐	Mushrooms	☐	Spinach

MEAT AND SEAFOOD

☐	Bacon	☐	Lamb	☐	Fish
☐	Beef	☐	Pork	☐	Crab
☐	Bison	☐	Rotisserie Chicken	☐	Lobster
☐	Chicken	☐	Sausage	☐	Scallops
☐	Deli meat	☐	Turkey	☐	Shrimp
☐	Ground Beef / Ground Turkey	☐	Oyster	☐	Mussels

DAIRY PRODUCTS

☐	Butter	☐	Eggs	☐	Sour Cream
☐	Cheese	☐	Greek Yogurt, full fat	☐	Ghee
☐	Cream Cheese	☐	Heavy Whipping Cream	☐	Mayo

PANTRY ITEMS

☐	Avocado oil	☐	Tea/Coffee	☐	Moon Cheese
☐	Beef Jerky	☐	Pork Rinds	☐	Low Carb Protein Bars
☐	Bone Broth	☐	Mayonnaise	☐	All Natural Peanut Butter
☐	Tuna, Salmon (canned)	☐	Low Carb Salad Dressing	☐	Stevia
☐	Coconut Butter	☐	Olive oil, extra virgin	☐	Almonds
☐	Coconut Oil	☐	Olives	☐	Spices
☐	Almond Milk	☐	Sweeteners	☐	Almond Flour

FROZEN / OTHER

☐		☐		☐	
☐		☐		☐	
☐		☐		☐	
☐		☐		☐	

Low Carb Shopping List

FRESH PRODUCE

MEAT AND SEAFOOD

DAIRY PRODUCTS

PANTRY ITEMS

FROZEN / OTHER

Meal Planner

GROCERY LIST

- ☐
- ☐
- ☐
- ☐
- ☐
- ☐
- ☐
- ☐
- ☐
- ☐
- ☐
- ☐
- ☐
- ☐
- ☐
- ☐
- ☐

MON

TUES

WED

THUR

FRI

SAT

SUN

Weight Loss *Journal*

MONDAY

TUESDAY

WEDNESDAY

THURSDAY

FRIDAY

SATURDAY

SUNDAY

WEEK OF:

DATE	WEIGHT LOSS ACTION PLAN

NOTES

My Weight Loss Routine

CREATING A ROUTINE FOR SUCCESS

WEIGHT LOSS SUCCESS: HABIT & ROUTINE TRACKER

DRINK LOTS OF WATER TODAY		TRACK TOTAL CARB INTAKE	

COMPLETE TOP 3 GOALS OF THE DAY

1
2
3

PLAN MY MEALS FOR THE DAY:

BREAKFAST	LUNCH	DINNER

DAILY TRACKER & TO DO LIST	ACCOMPLISHMENTS

NOTES

Daily Tracker

SLEEP TRACKER:

DATE _____

| RISE: | BEDTIME: | SLEEP (HRS): |

NOTES FOR THE DAY

EXERCISE / WORKOUT ROUTINE

TOP 6 PRIORITIES OF THE DAY

IN A STATE OF KETOSIS?

YES   NO   UNSURE

WATER INTAKE TRACKER

DAILY ENERGY LEVEL

HIGH   **MEDIUM**   **LOW**

BREAKFAST

FAT: CARBS: PROTEIN: CALORIES:

LUNCH

FAT: CARBS: PROTEIN: CALORIES:

DINNER

FAT: CARBS: PROTEIN: CALORIES:

SNACKS

FAT: CARBS: PROTEIN: CALORIES:

END OF THE DAY TOTAL OVERVIEW

CARBS   FAT   PROTEIN
CALORIES

Staying On Track

MY WEIGHT LOSS DIARY:

_____
_____
_____
_____

WATER TRACKER

LOW CARB SNACKS

NOTES & REMINDERS

DOODLE MY MOOD

BREAKFAST IDEAS

LUNCH IDEAS

DINNER IDEAS

Daily Tracker

SLEEP TRACKER:

DATE _____

RISE: _____

BEDTIME: _____

SLEEP (HRS): _____

NOTES FOR THE DAY

_____

_____

EXERCISE / WORKOUT ROUTINE

IN A STATE OF KETOSIS?

YES   NO   UNSURE

WATER INTAKE TRACKER

DAILY ENERGY LEVEL		
HIGH	**MEDIUM**	**LOW**

BREAKFAST

FAT: CARBS: PROTEIN: CALORIES:

LUNCH

FAT: CARBS: PROTEIN: CALORIES:

DINNER

FAT: CARBS: PROTEIN: CALORIES:

SNACKS

FAT: CARBS: PROTEIN: CALORIES:

TOP 6 PRIORITIES OF THE DAY

END OF THE DAY TOTAL OVERVIEW

CARBS   FAT   PROTEIN
CALORIES

Staying On Track

MY WEIGHT LOSS DIARY:

_____
_____
_____
_____

WATER TRACKER

LOW CARB SNACKS

NOTES & REMINDERS

DOODLE MY MOOD

BREAKFAST IDEAS

LUNCH IDEAS

DINNER IDEAS

Daily Tracker

SLEEP TRACKER:

DATE _____

RISE: _____   BEDTIME: _____   SLEEP (HRS): _____

NOTES FOR THE DAY

IN A STATE OF KETOSIS?

YES   NO   UNSURE

WATER INTAKE TRACKER

EXERCISE / WORKOUT ROUTINE

DAILY ENERGY LEVEL		
HIGH	**MEDIUM**	**LOW**

BREAKFAST

FAT: CARBS: PROTEIN: CALORIES:

LUNCH

FAT: CARBS: PROTEIN: CALORIES:

DINNER

FAT: CARBS: PROTEIN: CALORIES:

SNACKS

FAT: CARBS: PROTEIN: CALORIES:

TOP 6 PRIORITIES OF THE DAY

END OF THE DAY TOTAL OVERVIEW

CARBS   FAT   PROTEIN
CALORIES

Staying On Track

MY WEIGHT LOSS DIARY:

WATER TRACKER

LOW CARB SNACKS

NOTES & REMINDERS

DOODLE MY MOOD

BREAKFAST IDEAS

LUNCH IDEAS

DINNER IDEAS

Daily Tracker

SLEEP TRACKER:

DATE _____

 RISE: _____ | BEDTIME: _____ | SLEEP (HRS): _____

NOTES FOR THE DAY

_____

_____

_____

EXERCISE / WORKOUT ROUTINE

TOP 6 PRIORITIES OF THE DAY

IN A STATE OF KETOSIS?

YES   NO   UNSURE

WATER INTAKE TRACKER

DAILY ENERGY LEVEL

HIGH   **MEDIUM**   **LOW**

BREAKFAST

FAT: CARBS: PROTEIN: CALORIES:

LUNCH

FAT: CARBS: PROTEIN: CALORIES:

DINNER

FAT: CARBS: PROTEIN: CALORIES:

SNACKS

FAT: CARBS: PROTEIN: CALORIES:

END OF THE DAY TOTAL OVERVIEW

CARBS   FAT   PROTEIN
CALORIES

Staying On Track

MY WEIGHT LOSS DIARY:

_____
_____
_____
_____

WATER TRACKER

◇ ◇ ◇ ◇ ◇ ◇ ◇

LOW CARB SNACKS

NOTES & REMINDERS

_____
_____
_____
_____
_____
_____
_____
_____
_____
_____
_____

DOODLE MY MOOD

BREAKFAST IDEAS

LUNCH IDEAS

DINNER IDEAS

Daily Tracker

DATE _____

SLEEP TRACKER:

RISE: _____   BEDTIME: _____   SLEEP (HRS): _____

NOTES FOR THE DAY

_____

_____

_____

IN A STATE OF KETOSIS?

YES   NO   UNSURE

WATER INTAKE TRACKER

EXERCISE / WORKOUT ROUTINE

DAILY ENERGY LEVEL		
HIGH	**MEDIUM**	**LOW**

BREAKFAST

FAT: CARBS: PROTEIN: CALORIES:

LUNCH

FAT: CARBS: PROTEIN: CALORIES:

DINNER

FAT: CARBS: PROTEIN: CALORIES:

SNACKS

FAT: CARBS: PROTEIN: CALORIES:

TOP 6 PRIORITIES OF THE DAY

END OF THE DAY TOTAL OVERVIEW

CARBS   FAT   PROTEIN
CALORIES

Staying On Track

MY WEIGHT LOSS DIARY:

_____
_____
_____
_____

WATER TRACKER

LOW CARB SNACKS

NOTES & REMINDERS

DOODLE MY MOOD

BREAKFAST IDEAS

LUNCH IDEAS

DINNER IDEAS

Daily Tracker

SLEEP TRACKER:

DATE _____

 RISE: [_____]

🌙 BEDTIME: [_____]

 SLEEP (HRS): [_____]

NOTES FOR THE DAY

_____
_____
_____

EXERCISE / WORKOUT ROUTINE

IN A STATE OF KETOSIS?

YES   NO   UNSURE

WATER INTAKE TRACKER

💧 💧 💧 💧 💧 💧 💧 💧

DAILY ENERGY LEVEL		
HIGH	**MEDIUM**	**LOW**

BREAKFAST

FAT: CARBS: PROTEIN: CALORIES:

LUNCH

FAT: CARBS: PROTEIN: CALORIES:

DINNER

FAT: CARBS: PROTEIN: CALORIES:

SNACKS

FAT: CARBS: PROTEIN: CALORIES:

TOP 6 PRIORITIES OF THE DAY

○ _____ ○ _____
○ _____ ○ _____
○ _____ ○ _____

END OF THE DAY TOTAL OVERVIEW

CARBS   FAT   PROTEIN
CALORIES

Staying On Track

MY WEIGHT LOSS DIARY:

_____

_____

_____

_____

WATER TRACKER

NOTES & REMINDERS

DOODLE MY MOOD

LOW CARB SNACKS

BREAKFAST IDEAS

LUNCH IDEAS

DINNER IDEAS

Daily Tracker

SLEEP TRACKER:

DATE _____

☀	RISE:

🌙 | BEDTIME: |

 | SLEEP (HRS): |

NOTES FOR THE DAY

_____

_____

_____

EXERCISE / WORKOUT ROUTINE

IN A STATE OF KETOSIS?

YES   NO   UNSURE

WATER INTAKE TRACKER

DAILY ENERGY LEVEL

HIGH   **MEDIUM**   **LOW**

BREAKFAST

FAT: CARBS: PROTEIN: CALORIES:

LUNCH

FAT: CARBS: PROTEIN: CALORIES:

DINNER

FAT: CARBS: PROTEIN: CALORIES:

SNACKS

FAT: CARBS: PROTEIN: CALORIES:

TOP 6 PRIORITIES OF THE DAY

END OF THE DAY TOTAL OVERVIEW

CARBS   FAT   PROTEIN
CALORIES

Staying On Track

MY WEIGHT LOSS DIARY:

_____

_____

_____

_____

WATER TRACKER

LOW CARB SNACKS

NOTES & REMINDERS

_____

_____

_____

_____

_____

_____

_____

_____

_____

_____

_____

DOODLE MY MOOD

BREAKFAST IDEAS

LUNCH IDEAS

DINNER IDEAS

Keto Go To Meals

BREAKFAST	LUNCH	DINNER	SNACKS
BREAKFAST	LUNCH	DINNER	SNACKS
BREAKFAST	LUNCH	DINNER	SNACKS
BREAKFAST	LUNCH	DINNER	SNACKS
BREAKFAST	LUNCH	DINNER	SNACKS
BREAKFAST	LUNCH	DINNER	SNACKS
BREAKFAST	LUNCH	DINNER	SNACKS

WEEK OF:

KETO *Meal* LOG BOOK

	BREAKFAST	LUNCH	DINNER	SNACKS
MONDAY				
TUESDAY				
WEDNESDAY				
THURSDAY				
FRIDAY				
SATURDAY				
SUNDAY				

Weekly Fasting *Tracker*

Week Of: _____

MONDAY

	12	1	2	3	4	5	6	7	8	9	10	11	12	1	2	3	4	5	6	7	8	9	10	11
Goal	12	1	2	3	4	5	6	7	8	9	10	11	12	1	2	3	4	5	6	7	8	9	10	11
Actual	12	1	2	3	4	5	6	7	8	9	10	11	12	1	2	3	4	5	6	7	8	9	10	11

TUESDAY

	12	1	2	3	4	5	6	7	8	9	10	11	12	1	2	3	4	5	6	7	8	9	10	11
Goal	12	1	2	3	4	5	6	7	8	9	10	11	12	1	2	3	4	5	6	7	8	9	10	11
Actual	12	1	2	3	4	5	6	7	8	9	10	11	12	1	2	3	4	5	6	7	8	9	10	11

WEDNESDAY

	12	1	2	3	4	5	6	7	8	9	10	11	12	1	2	3	4	5	6	7	8	9	10	11
Goal	12	1	2	3	4	5	6	7	8	9	10	11	12	1	2	3	4	5	6	7	8	9	10	11
Actual	12	1	2	3	4	5	6	7	8	9	10	11	12	1	2	3	4	5	6	7	8	9	10	11

THURSDAY

	12	1	2	3	4	5	6	7	8	9	10	11	12	1	2	3	4	5	6	7	8	9	10	11
Goal	12	1	2	3	4	5	6	7	8	9	10	11	12	1	2	3	4	5	6	7	8	9	10	11
Actual	12	1	2	3	4	5	6	7	8	9	10	11	12	1	2	3	4	5	6	7	8	9	10	11

FRIDAY

	12	1	2	3	4	5	6	7	8	9	10	11	12	1	2	3	4	5	6	7	8	9	10	11
Goal	12	1	2	3	4	5	6	7	8	9	10	11	12	1	2	3	4	5	6	7	8	9	10	11
Actual	12	1	2	3	4	5	6	7	8	9	10	11	12	1	2	3	4	5	6	7	8	9	10	11

SATURDAY

	12	1	2	3	4	5	6	7	8	9	10	11	12	1	2	3	4	5	6	7	8	9	10	11
Goal	12	1	2	3	4	5	6	7	8	9	10	11	12	1	2	3	4	5	6	7	8	9	10	11
Actual	12	1	2	3	4	5	6	7	8	9	10	11	12	1	2	3	4	5	6	7	8	9	10	11

SUNDAY

	12	1	2	3	4	5	6	7	8	9	10	11	12	1	2	3	4	5	6	7	8	9	10	11
Goal	12	1	2	3	4	5	6	7	8	9	10	11	12	1	2	3	4	5	6	7	8	9	10	11
Actual	12	1	2	3	4	5	6	7	8	9	10	11	12	1	2	3	4	5	6	7	8	9	10	11

Weekly Progress

Monday

Tuesday

Wednesday

Thursday

Friday

Saturday

Sunday

Notes

Low Carb Grocery Ideas

FRESH PRODUCE

☐ Asparagus	☐ Cauliflower	☐ Onions
☐ Avocado	☐ Celery	☐ Radishes
☐ Bell Peppers	☐ Cucumber	☐ Salad Mix
☐ Berries	☐ Eggplant	☐ Squash
☐ Broccoli	☐ Fennel	☐ Tomatoes
☐ Brussel Sprouts	☐ Garlic	☐ Bok Choi
☐ Cabbage	☐ Green Beans	☐ Chives
☐ Carrots	☐ Mushrooms	☐ Spinach

MEAT AND SEAFOOD

☐ Bacon	☐ Lamb	☐ Fish
☐ Beef	☐ Pork	☐ Crab
☐ Bison	☐ Rotisserie Chicken	☐ Lobster
☐ Chicken	☐ Sausage	☐ Scallops
☐ Deli meat	☐ Turkey	☐ Shrimp
☐ Ground Beef / Ground Turkey	☐ Oyster	☐ Mussels

DAIRY PRODUCTS

☐ Butter	☐ Eggs	☐ Sour Cream
☐ Cheese	☐ Greek Yogurt, full fat	☐ Ghee
☐ Cream Cheese	☐ Heavy Whipping Cream	☐ Mayo

PANTRY ITEMS

☐ Avocado oil	☐ Tea/Coffee	☐ Moon Cheese
☐ Beef Jerky	☐ Pork Rinds	☐ Low Carb Protein Bars
☐ Bone Broth	☐ Mayonnaise	☐ All Natural Peanut Butter
☐ Tuna, Salmon (canned)	☐ Low Carb Salad Dressing	☐ Stevia
☐ Coconut Butter	☐ Olive oil, extra virgin	☐ Almonds
☐ Coconut Oil	☐ Olives	☐ Spices
☐ Almond Milk	☐ Sweeteners	☐ Almond Flour

FROZEN / OTHER

☐	☐	☐
☐	☐	☐
☐	☐	☐

Low Carb Shopping List

FRESH PRODUCE

MEAT AND SEAFOOD

DAIRY PRODUCTS

PANTRY ITEMS

FROZEN / OTHER

Meal Planner

WEEK OF

GROCERY LIST

- ☐
- ☐
- ☐
- ☐
- ☐
- ☐
- ☐
- ☐
- ☐
- ☐
- ☐
- ☐
- ☐
- ☐
- ☐
- ☐
- ☐
- ☐

MON

TUES

WED

THUR

FRI

SAT

SUN

Weight Loss *Journal*

MONDAY

TUESDAY

WEDNESDAY

THURSDAY

FRIDAY

SATURDAY

SUNDAY

WEEK OF:

DATE	WEIGHT LOSS ACTION PLAN

NOTES

My Weight Loss Routine

WEIGHT LOSS SUCCESS: HABIT & ROUTINE TRACKER

DRINK LOTS OF WATER TODAY	◯	TRACK TOTAL CARB INTAKE	◯

COMPLETE TOP 3 GOALS OF THE DAY

1
2
3

PLAN MY MEALS FOR THE DAY:

BREAKFAST	LUNCH	DINNER

DAILY TRACKER & TO DO LIST   ACCOMPLISHMENTS

◯
◯
◯
◯
◯

NOTES

Daily Tracker

SLEEP TRACKER:

DATE _____

☀ RISE: _____   ☾ᶻᶻᶻ BEDTIME: _____   💭ᶻᶻᶻ SLEEP (HRS): _____

NOTES FOR THE DAY

_____
_____
_____

EXERCISE / WORKOUT ROUTINE

IN A STATE OF KETOSIS?

YES   NO   UNSURE

WATER INTAKE TRACKER

💧 💧 💧 💧 💧 💧 💧

DAILY ENERGY LEVEL		
HIGH	**MEDIUM**	**LOW**

BREAKFAST

FAT: CARBS: PROTEIN: CALORIES:

LUNCH

FAT: CARBS: PROTEIN: CALORIES:

DINNER

FAT: CARBS: PROTEIN: CALORIES:

SNACKS

FAT: CARBS: PROTEIN: CALORIES:

TOP 6 PRIORITIES OF THE DAY

○ _____   ○ _____
○ _____   ○ _____
○ _____   ○ _____

END OF THE DAY TOTAL OVERVIEW

CARBS   FAT   PROTEIN
CALORIES

Staying On Track

MY WEIGHT LOSS DIARY:

WATER TRACKER

LOW CARB SNACKS

NOTES & REMINDERS

DOODLE MY MOOD

BREAKFAST IDEAS

LUNCH IDEAS

DINNER IDEAS

Daily Tracker

SLEEP TRACKER:

DATE _____

	RISE:		BEDTIME:		SLEEP (HRS):

NOTES FOR THE DAY

_____

_____

_____

EXERCISE / WORKOUT ROUTINE

TOP 6 PRIORITIES OF THE DAY

- ○ _____ ○ _____
- ○ _____ ○ _____
- ○ _____ ○ _____

IN A STATE OF KETOSIS?

YES   NO   UNSURE

WATER INTAKE TRACKER

DAILY ENERGY LEVEL

HIGH	MEDIUM	LOW

BREAKFAST

FAT: CARBS: PROTEIN: CALORIES:

LUNCH

FAT: CARBS: PROTEIN: CALORIES:

DINNER

FAT: CARBS: PROTEIN: CALORIES:

SNACKS

FAT: CARBS: PROTEIN: CALORIES:

END OF THE DAY TOTAL OVERVIEW

CARBS CALORIES	FAT	PROTEIN

Staying On Track

MY WEIGHT LOSS DIARY:

_____
_____
_____
_____

WATER TRACKER

LOW CARB SNACKS

NOTES & REMINDERS

DOODLE MY MOOD

BREAKFAST IDEAS

LUNCH IDEAS

DINNER IDEAS

Daily Tracker

SLEEP TRACKER:

DATE _____

☀ | RISE: | 🌙 | BEDTIME: | 💭 | SLEEP (HRS):

NOTES FOR THE DAY

_____

_____

_____

EXERCISE / WORKOUT ROUTINE

IN A STATE OF KETOSIS?

YES   NO   UNSURE

WATER INTAKE TRACKER

💧 💧 💧 💧 💧 💧 💧

DAILY ENERGY LEVEL		
HIGH	**MEDIUM**	**LOW**

BREAKFAST

FAT: CARBS: PROTEIN: CALORIES:

LUNCH

FAT: CARBS: PROTEIN: CALORIES:

DINNER

FAT: CARBS: PROTEIN: CALORIES:

SNACKS

FAT: CARBS: PROTEIN: CALORIES:

TOP 6 PRIORITIES OF THE DAY

○ _____   ○ _____

○ _____   ○ _____

○ _____   ○ _____

END OF THE DAY TOTAL OVERVIEW

CARBS   FAT   PROTEIN
CALORIES

Staying On Track

MY WEIGHT LOSS DIARY:

_____

_____

_____

_____

WATER TRACKER

LOW CARB SNACKS

NOTES & REMINDERS

DOODLE MY MOOD

BREAKFAST IDEAS

LUNCH IDEAS

DINNER IDEAS

Daily Tracker

SLEEP TRACKER:

DATE _____

RISE: _____   BEDTIME: _____   SLEEP (HRS): _____

NOTES FOR THE DAY

_____
_____
_____

IN A STATE OF KETOSIS?

YES   NO   UNSURE

WATER INTAKE TRACKER

EXERCISE / WORKOUT ROUTINE

DAILY ENERGY LEVEL		
HIGH	**MEDIUM**	**LOW**

BREAKFAST

FAT: CARBS: PROTEIN: CALORIES:

LUNCH

FAT: CARBS: PROTEIN: CALORIES:

DINNER

FAT: CARBS: PROTEIN: CALORIES:

SNACKS

FAT: CARBS: PROTEIN: CALORIES:

TOP 6 PRIORITIES OF THE DAY

END OF THE DAY TOTAL OVERVIEW

CARBS   FAT   PROTEIN
CALORIES

Staying On Track

MY WEIGHT LOSS DIARY:

WATER TRACKER

LOW CARB SNACKS

NOTES & REMINDERS

DOODLE MY MOOD

BREAKFAST IDEAS

LUNCH IDEAS

DINNER IDEAS

Daily Tracker

SLEEP TRACKER:

DATE _____

☀ | RISE:

🌙 | BEDTIME:

💭 | SLEEP (HRS):

NOTES FOR THE DAY

_____

_____

_____

EXERCISE / WORKOUT ROUTINE

TOP 6 PRIORITIES OF THE DAY

- ○ _____ ○ _____
- ○ _____ ○ _____
- ○ _____ ○ _____

IN A STATE OF KETOSIS?

YES   NO   UNSURE

WATER INTAKE TRACKER

💧 💧 💧 💧 💧 💧 💧

DAILY ENERGY LEVEL		
HIGH	**MEDIUM**	**LOW**

BREAKFAST

FAT: CARBS: PROTEIN: CALORIES:

LUNCH

FAT: CARBS: PROTEIN: CALORIES:

DINNER

FAT: CARBS: PROTEIN: CALORIES:

SNACKS

FAT: CARBS: PROTEIN: CALORIES:

END OF THE DAY TOTAL OVERVIEW

CARBS   FAT   PROTEIN
CALORIES

Staying On Track

MY WEIGHT LOSS DIARY:

_____

_____

_____

_____

WATER TRACKER

LOW CARB SNACKS

NOTES & REMINDERS

DOODLE MY MOOD

BREAKFAST IDEAS

LUNCH IDEAS

DINNER IDEAS

Daily Tracker

SLEEP TRACKER:

DATE _____

☀ | RISE: | 🌙 z,z | BEDTIME: | 💭 z²z | SLEEP (HRS): |

NOTES FOR THE DAY

_____
_____
_____

EXERCISE / WORKOUT ROUTINE

IN A STATE OF KETOSIS?

YES   NO   UNSURE

WATER INTAKE TRACKER

💧 💧 💧 💧 💧 💧 💧 💧

DAILY ENERGY LEVEL		
HIGH	**MEDIUM**	**LOW**

BREAKFAST

FAT: CARBS: PROTEIN: CALORIES:

LUNCH

FAT: CARBS: PROTEIN: CALORIES:

DINNER

FAT: CARBS: PROTEIN: CALORIES:

SNACKS

FAT: CARBS: PROTEIN: CALORIES:

TOP 6 PRIORITIES OF THE DAY

● _____   ● _____

● _____   ● _____

● _____   ● _____

END OF THE DAY TOTAL OVERVIEW

CARBS   FAT   PROTEIN
CALORIES

Staying On Track

MY WEIGHT LOSS DIARY:

_____
_____
_____
_____

WATER TRACKER

LOW CARB SNACKS

NOTES & REMINDERS

_____
_____
_____
_____
_____
_____
_____
_____

DOODLE MY MOOD

BREAKFAST IDEAS

LUNCH IDEAS

DINNER IDEAS

Daily Tracker

SLEEP TRACKER:

DATE _____

☀ RISE: _____   🌙 BEDTIME: _____   💭 SLEEP (HRS): _____

NOTES FOR THE DAY

_____

_____

_____

EXERCISE / WORKOUT ROUTINE

IN A STATE OF KETOSIS?

YES   NO   UNSURE

WATER INTAKE TRACKER

💧 💧 💧 💧 💧 💧 💧

DAILY ENERGY LEVEL		
HIGH	**MEDIUM**	**LOW**

BREAKFAST

FAT: CARBS: PROTEIN: CALORIES:

LUNCH

FAT: CARBS: PROTEIN: CALORIES:

DINNER

FAT: CARBS: PROTEIN: CALORIES:

SNACKS

FAT: CARBS: PROTEIN: CALORIES:

TOP 6 PRIORITIES OF THE DAY

○ _____   ○ _____

○ _____   ○ _____

○ _____   ○ _____

END OF THE DAY TOTAL OVERVIEW

CARBS   FAT   PROTEIN
CALORIES

Staying On Track

MY WEIGHT LOSS DIARY:

_____
_____
_____
_____

WATER TRACKER

NOTES & REMINDERS

DOODLE MY MOOD

LOW CARB SNACKS

BREAKFAST IDEAS

LUNCH IDEAS

DINNER IDEAS

Keto Go To Meals

FAVORITE KETO FRIENDLY MEALS

BREAKFAST	LUNCH	DINNER	SNACKS
BREAKFAST	LUNCH	DINNER	SNACKS
BREAKFAST	LUNCH	DINNER	SNACKS
BREAKFAST	LUNCH	DINNER	SNACKS
BREAKFAST	LUNCH	DINNER	SNACKS
BREAKFAST	LUNCH	DINNER	SNACKS
BREAKFAST	LUNCH	DINNER	SNACKS

WEEK OF:

KETO *Meal* LOG BOOK

	BREAKFAST	LUNCH	DINNER	SNACKS
MONDAY				
TUESDAY				
WEDNESDAY				
THURSDAY				
FRIDAY				
SATURDAY				
SUNDAY				

Weekly Fasting Tracker

Week Of: _____

MONDAY

	12	1	2	3	4	5	6	7	8	9	10	11	12	1	2	3	4	5	6	7	8	9	10	11
Goal	12	1	2	3	4	5	6	7	8	9	10	11	12	1	2	3	4	5	6	7	8	9	10	11
Actual	12	1	2	3	4	5	6	7	8	9	10	11	12	1	2	3	4	5	6	7	8	9	10	11

TUESDAY

	12	1	2	3	4	5	6	7	8	9	10	11	12	1	2	3	4	5	6	7	8	9	10	11
Goal	12	1	2	3	4	5	6	7	8	9	10	11	12	1	2	3	4	5	6	7	8	9	10	11
Actual	12	1	2	3	4	5	6	7	8	9	10	11	12	1	2	3	4	5	6	7	8	9	10	11

WEDNESDAY

	12	1	2	3	4	5	6	7	8	9	10	11	12	1	2	3	4	5	6	7	8	9	10	11
Goal	12	1	2	3	4	5	6	7	8	9	10	11	12	1	2	3	4	5	6	7	8	9	10	11
Actual	12	1	2	3	4	5	6	7	8	9	10	11	12	1	2	3	4	5	6	7	8	9	10	11

THURSDAY

	12	1	2	3	4	5	6	7	8	9	10	11	12	1	2	3	4	5	6	7	8	9	10	11
Goal	12	1	2	3	4	5	6	7	8	9	10	11	12	1	2	3	4	5	6	7	8	9	10	11
Actual	12	1	2	3	4	5	6	7	8	9	10	11	12	1	2	3	4	5	6	7	8	9	10	11

FRIDAY

	12	1	2	3	4	5	6	7	8	9	10	11	12	1	2	3	4	5	6	7	8	9	10	11
Goal	12	1	2	3	4	5	6	7	8	9	10	11	12	1	2	3	4	5	6	7	8	9	10	11
Actual	12	1	2	3	4	5	6	7	8	9	10	11	12	1	2	3	4	5	6	7	8	9	10	11

SATURDAY

	12	1	2	3	4	5	6	7	8	9	10	11	12	1	2	3	4	5	6	7	8	9	10	11
Goal	12	1	2	3	4	5	6	7	8	9	10	11	12	1	2	3	4	5	6	7	8	9	10	11
Actual	12	1	2	3	4	5	6	7	8	9	10	11	12	1	2	3	4	5	6	7	8	9	10	11

SUNDAY

	12	1	2	3	4	5	6	7	8	9	10	11	12	1	2	3	4	5	6	7	8	9	10	11
Goal	12	1	2	3	4	5	6	7	8	9	10	11	12	1	2	3	4	5	6	7	8	9	10	11
Actual	12	1	2	3	4	5	6	7	8	9	10	11	12	1	2	3	4	5	6	7	8	9	10	11

Weekly Progress

WEEK OF : _____

Monday

Tuesday

Wednesday

Thursday

Friday

Saturday

Sunday

Notes

Low Carb *Grocery Ideas*

FRESH PRODUCE

☐ Asparagus	☐ Cauliflower	☐ Onions
☐ Avocado	☐ Celery	☐ Radishes
☐ Bell Peppers	☐ Cucumber	☐ Salad Mix
☐ Berries	☐ Eggplant	☐ Squash
☐ Broccoli	☐ Fennel	☐ Tomatoes
☐ Brussel Sprouts	☐ Garlic	☐ Bok Choi
☐ Cabbage	☐ Green Beans	☐ Chives
☐ Carrots	☐ Mushrooms	☐ Spinach

MEAT AND SEAFOOD

☐ Bacon	☐ Lamb	☐ Fish
☐ Beef	☐ Pork	☐ Crab
☐ Bison	☐ Rotisserie Chicken	☐ Lobster
☐ Chicken	☐ Sausage	☐ Scallops
☐ Deli meat	☐ Turkey	☐ Shrimp
☐ Ground Beef / Ground Turkey	☐ Oyster	☐ Mussels

DAIRY PRODUCTS

☐ Butter	☐ Eggs	☐ Sour Cream
☐ Cheese	☐ Greek Yogurt, full fat	☐ Ghee
☐ Cream Cheese	☐ Heavy Whipping Cream	☐ Mayo

PANTRY ITEMS

☐ Avocado oil	☐ Tea/Coffee	☐ Moon Cheese
☐ Beef Jerky	☐ Pork Rinds	☐ Low Carb Protein Bars
☐ Bone Broth	☐ Mayonnaise	☐ All Natural Peanut Butter
☐ Tuna, Salmon (canned)	☐ Low Carb Salad Dressing	☐ Stevia
☐ Coconut Butter	☐ Olive oil, extra virgin	☐ Almonds
☐ Coconut Oil	☐ Olives	☐ Spices
☐ Almond Milk	☐ Sweeteners	☐ Almond Flour

FROZEN / OTHER

☐	☐	☐
☐	☐	☐
☐	☐	☐
☐	☐	☐

Keto Grocery Inventory

DATE: _____

QTY	PRODUCE

QTY	MEAT & FISH

QTY	FROZEN FOODS

QTY	DAIRY

QTY	PANTRY

QTY	OTHER/MISC.

Low Carb Shopping List

FRESH PRODUCE

MEAT AND SEAFOOD

DAIRY PRODUCTS

PANTRY ITEMS

FROZEN / OTHER

Meal Planner

GROCERY LIST

- [ ]
- [ ]
- [ ]
- [ ]
- [ ]
- [ ]
- [ ]
- [ ]
- [ ]
- [ ]
- [ ]
- [ ]
- [ ]
- [ ]
- [ ]

MON

TUES

WED

THUR

FRI

SAT

SUN

Weight Loss *Journal*

MONDAY

TUESDAY

WEDNESDAY

THURSDAY

FRIDAY

SATURDAY

SUNDAY

WEEK OF:

DATE	WEIGHT LOSS ACTION PLAN

NOTES

My Weight Loss Routine

CREATING A ROUTINE FOR SUCCESS

WEIGHT LOSS SUCCESS: HABIT & ROUTINE TRACKER

DRINK LOTS OF WATER TODAY	TRACK TOTAL CARB INTAKE

COMPLETE TOP 3 GOALS OF THE DAY

1

2

3

PLAN MY MEALS FOR THE DAY:

BREAKFAST	LUNCH	DINNER

DAILY TRACKER & TO DO LIST	ACCOMPLISHMENTS

NOTES

Daily Tracker

SLEEP TRACKER:

DATE _____

☀ RISE: _____   🌙 BEDTIME: _____   💤 SLEEP (HRS): _____

NOTES FOR THE DAY

_____

_____

_____

EXERCISE / WORKOUT ROUTINE

IN A STATE OF KETOSIS?

YES   NO   UNSURE

WATER INTAKE TRACKER

💧 💧 💧 💧 💧 💧 💧 💧

DAILY ENERGY LEVEL

HIGH   **MEDIUM**   **LOW**

BREAKFAST

FAT: CARBS: PROTEIN: CALORIES:

LUNCH

FAT: CARBS: PROTEIN: CALORIES:

DINNER

FAT: CARBS: PROTEIN: CALORIES:

SNACKS

FAT: CARBS: PROTEIN: CALORIES:

TOP 6 PRIORITIES OF THE DAY

● _____   ● _____

● _____   ● _____

● _____   ● _____

END OF THE DAY TOTAL OVERVIEW

CARBS   FAT   PROTEIN
CALORIES

_____   _____   _____

Staying On Track

MY WEIGHT LOSS DIARY:

_____

_____

_____

_____

WATER TRACKER

LOW CARB SNACKS

NOTES & REMINDERS

DOODLE MY MOOD

BREAKFAST IDEAS

LUNCH IDEAS

DINNER IDEAS

Daily Tracker

SLEEP TRACKER:

DATE _____

RISE: | BEDTIME: | SLEEP (HRS):

NOTES FOR THE DAY

IN A STATE OF KETOSIS?

YES   NO   UNSURE

WATER INTAKE TRACKER

EXERCISE / WORKOUT ROUTINE

DAILY ENERGY LEVEL		
HIGH	**MEDIUM**	**LOW**

BREAKFAST

FAT: CARBS: PROTEIN: CALORIES:

LUNCH

FAT: CARBS: PROTEIN: CALORIES:

DINNER

FAT: CARBS: PROTEIN: CALORIES:

SNACKS

FAT: CARBS: PROTEIN: CALORIES:

TOP 6 PRIORITIES OF THE DAY

END OF THE DAY TOTAL OVERVIEW

CARBS   FAT   PROTEIN
CALORIES

Staying On Track

MY WEIGHT LOSS DIARY:

_____
_____
_____
_____

WATER TRACKER

LOW CARB SNACKS

NOTES & REMINDERS

DOODLE MY MOOD

BREAKFAST IDEAS

LUNCH IDEAS

DINNER IDEAS

Keto Go To Meals

FAVORITE KETO FRIENDLY MEALS

BREAKFAST	LUNCH	DINNER	SNACKS
BREAKFAST	LUNCH	DINNER	SNACKS
BREAKFAST	LUNCH	DINNER	SNACKS
BREAKFAST	LUNCH	DINNER	SNACKS
BREAKFAST	LUNCH	DINNER	SNACKS
BREAKFAST	LUNCH	DINNER	SNACKS
BREAKFAST	LUNCH	DINNER	SNACKS

KETO *Meal* LOG BOOK

WEEK OF:

	BREAKFAST	LUNCH	DINNER	SNACKS
MONDAY				
TUESDAY				
WEDNESDAY				
THURSDAY				
FRIDAY				
SATURDAY				
SUNDAY				

Weekly Fasting Tracker

Week Of: _____

MONDAY

Goal	12	1	2	3	4	5	6	7	8	9	10	11	12	1	2	3	4	5	6	7	8	9	10	11
Actual	12	1	2	3	4	5	6	7	8	9	10	11	12	1	2	3	4	5	6	7	8	9	10	11

TUESDAY

Goal	12	1	2	3	4	5	6	7	8	9	10	11	12	1	2	3	4	5	6	7	8	9	10	11
Actual	12	1	2	3	4	5	6	7	8	9	10	11	12	1	2	3	4	5	6	7	8	9	10	11

WEDNESDAY

Goal	12	1	2	3	4	5	6	7	8	9	10	11	12	1	2	3	4	5	6	7	8	9	10	11
Actual	12	1	2	3	4	5	6	7	8	9	10	11	12	1	2	3	4	5	6	7	8	9	10	11

THURSDAY

Goal	12	1	2	3	4	5	6	7	8	9	10	11	12	1	2	3	4	5	6	7	8	9	10	11
Actual	12	1	2	3	4	5	6	7	8	9	10	11	12	1	2	3	4	5	6	7	8	9	10	11

FRIDAY

Goal	12	1	2	3	4	5	6	7	8	9	10	11	12	1	2	3	4	5	6	7	8	9	10	11
Actual	12	1	2	3	4	5	6	7	8	9	10	11	12	1	2	3	4	5	6	7	8	9	10	11

SATURDAY

Goal	12	1	2	3	4	5	6	7	8	9	10	11	12	1	2	3	4	5	6	7	8	9	10	11
Actual	12	1	2	3	4	5	6	7	8	9	10	11	12	1	2	3	4	5	6	7	8	9	10	11

SUNDAY

Goal	12	1	2	3	4	5	6	7	8	9	10	11	12	1	2	3	4	5	6	7	8	9	10	11
Actual	12	1	2	3	4	5	6	7	8	9	10	11	12	1	2	3	4	5	6	7	8	9	10	11

Weekly Progress

WEEK OF : _____

Monday

Tuesday

Wednesday

Thursday

Friday

Saturday

Sunday

Notes

Intermittent *Fasting Log*

WEEK OF:

	START TIME	END TIME	TOTAL FAST HRS
M	:	:	:
T	:	:	:
W	:	:	:
T	:	:	:
F	:	:	:
S	:	:	:
S	:	:	:

WEEK OF:

	START TIME	END TIME	TOTAL FAST HRS
M	:	:	:
T	:	:	:
W	:	:	:
T	:	:	:
F	:	:	:
S	:	:	:
S	:	:	:

WEEK OF:

	START TIME	END TIME	TOTAL FAST HRS
M	:	:	:
T	:	:	:
W	:	:	:
T	:	:	:
F	:	:	:
S	:	:	:
S	:	:	:

WEEK OF:

	START TIME	END TIME	TOTAL FAST HRS
M	:	:	:
T	:	:	:
W	:	:	:
T	:	:	:
F	:	:	:
S	:	:	:
S	:	:	:

WEEK OF:

	START TIME	END TIME	TOTAL FAST HRS
M	:	:	:
T	:	:	:
W	:	:	:
T	:	:	:
F	:	:	:
S	:	:	:
S	:	:	:

WEEK OF:

	START TIME	END TIME	TOTAL FAST HRS
M	:	:	:
T	:	:	:
W	:	:	:
T	:	:	:
F	:	:	:
S	:	:	:
S	:	:	:

MILESTONES & ACCOMPLISHMENTS

NOTES & REFLECTIONS

Monthly Progress *Tracker*

| JAN | FEB | MAR | APR | MAY | JUN | JUL | AUG | SEP | OCT | NOV | DEC |

MON	TUE	WED	THU	FRI	SAT	SUN

WEIGHT LOSS MILESTONE TRACKER

CHEAT DAY TRACKER

WEEKLY DIET SUCCESS TRACKER & NOTES

Goals & Accomplishments

Month | JAN FEB MAR APR MAY JUN JUL AUG SEP OCT NOV DEC

THIS MONTH'S GOALS

ACTION PLAN

M T W T F S S

☐☐☐☐☐☐☐
☐☐☐☐☐☐☐
☐☐☐☐☐☐☐
☐☐☐☐☐☐☐
☐☐☐☐☐☐☐

NOTES:

WEEKLY GOALS

M

T

W

T

F

S

S

THOUGHTS

MEALS:	BREAKFAST	LUNCH	DINNER	SNACKS
M				
T				
W				
T				
F				
S				
S				

30 Days of Keto

STARTING WEIGHT:

DAY 30 WEIGHT:

(1) (2) (3) (4) (5) (6) (7) (8) (9) (10)

LBS LOST:

INCHES LOST:

(11) (12) (13) (14) (15) (16) (17) (18) (19) (20)

LBS LOST:

INCHES LOST:

(21) (22) (23) (24) (25) (26) (27) (28) (29) (30)

LBS LOST:

INCHES LOST:

TOTAL WEIGHT LOST:

TOTAL INCHES LOST:

NOTES:

PERSONAL ACCOMPLISHMENTS:

THOUGHTS & REFLECTIONS:

Weight Loss Tracker

MONTHLY GOAL

DATE:

BUST					
WAIST					
HIPS					
BICEP					
THIGH					
CALF					
WEIGHT					

TOTAL WEIGHT LOSS >>

Keto Recipe

RECIPE NAME:

	Keto	Low Carb	Paleo	Vegetarian	Vegan	Dairy Free	Gluten Free
	☐	☐	☐	☐	☐	☐	☐

QTY	INGREDIENTS	RECIPE INSTRUCTIONS

NOTES & RECIPE REVIEW

Serves	
Prep Time	
Cook Time	
Tools	
Temp	

Total	Carbs	Fat	Protein	Cals

Keto Recipe

RECIPE NAME:

	Keto	Low Carb	Paleo	Vegetarian	Vegan	Dairy Free	Gluten Free
	☐	☐	☐	☐	☐	☐	☐

QTY	INGREDIENTS

RECIPE INSTRUCTIONS

NOTES & RECIPE REVIEW

Serves	
Prep Time	
Cook Time	
Tools	
Temp	

Total	Carbs	Fat	Protein	Cals

Keto Recipe

RECIPE NAME:

Keto	Low Carb	Paleo	Vegetarian	Vegan	Dairy Free	Gluten Free
☐	☐	☐	☐	☐	☐	☐

QTY	INGREDIENTS

RECIPE INSTRUCTIONS

NOTES & RECIPE REVIEW

Serves	
Prep Time	
Cook Time	
Tools	
Temp	

Total	Carbs	Fat	Protein	Cals

Keto Recipe

RECIPE NAME:

_____

Keto	Low Carb	Paleo	Vegetarian	Vegan	Dairy Free	Gluten Free
☐	☐	☐	☐	☐	☐	☐

QTY	INGREDIENTS	RECIPE INSTRUCTIONS

NOTES & RECIPE REVIEW

Serves	
Prep Time	
Cook Time	
Tools	
Temp	

Total	Carbs	Fat	Protein	Cals

Keto Recipe

RECIPE NAME:

Keto	Low Carb	Paleo	Vegetarian	Vegan	Dairy Free	Gluten Free
☐	☐	☐	☐	☐	☐	☐

QTY	INGREDIENTS	RECIPE INSTRUCTIONS

NOTES & RECIPE REVIEW

Serves	
Prep Time	
Cook Time	
Tools	
Temp	

Total	Carbs	Fat	Protein	Cals

Keto Recipe

RECIPE NAME:

_____

Keto	Low Carb	Paleo	Vegetarian	Vegan	Dairy Free	Gluten Free
☐	☐	☐	☐	☐	☐	☐

QTY	INGREDIENTS

RECIPE INSTRUCTIONS

NOTES & RECIPE REVIEW

Serves	
Prep Time	
Cook Time	
Tools	
Temp	

Total	Carbs	Fat	Protein	Cals

Keto Recipe

RECIPE NAME:

Keto	Low Carb	Paleo	Vegetarian	Vegan	Dairy Free	Gluten Free
☐	☐	☐	☐	☐	☐	☐

QTY	INGREDIENTS	RECIPE INSTRUCTIONS

NOTES & RECIPE REVIEW

Serves	
Prep Time	
Cook Time	
Tools	
Temp	

Total	Carbs	Fat	Protein	Cals

Keto Recipe

RECIPE NAME:

_____

Keto	Low Carb	Paleo	Vegetarian	Vegan	Dairy Free	Gluten Free
☐	☐	☐	☐	☐	☐	☐

QTY	INGREDIENTS	RECIPE INSTRUCTIONS

NOTES & RECIPE REVIEW

Serves	
Prep Time	
Cook Time	
Tools	
Temp	

Total	Carbs	Fat	Protein	Cals

Printed in Great Britain
by Amazon